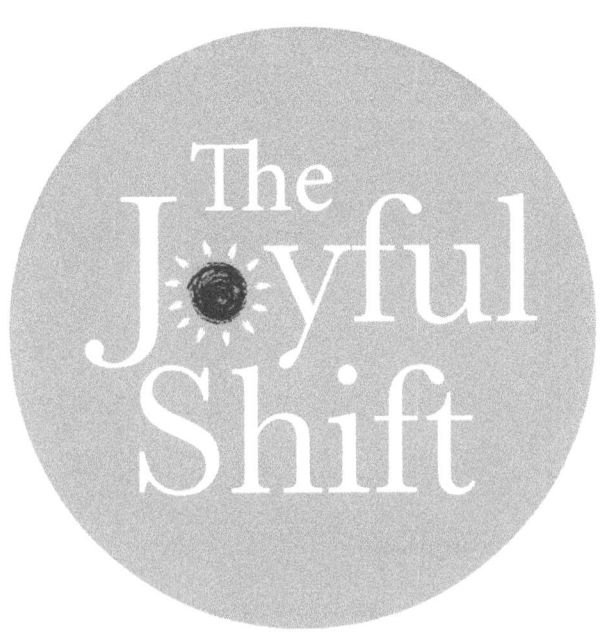

The J☀yful Shift

12 GUIDED LESSONS
TO INFUSE YOUR LIFE WITH
HAPPINESS AND PEACE

ALISON ANDERSON

First Edition

Cover and interior design by Claire Brown

This is a work of creative nonfiction. Some parts have been fictionalized in varying degrees, for various purposes.

ISBN 979-8-218-38250-6

Published by Alison Anderson

Kaysville, Utah 84037

Joyfulshiftbook@yahoo.com

For Eric. Who has taught me to open my eyes,
embrace every moment, and live with purpose.

Contents

Introduction..1

PART 1: Accept Yourself...7

Chapter 1: Practice Authenticity..9
Chapter 2: Establish Core Character................................19
Chapter 3: Value Imperfections.......................................29
Chapter 4: Get Curious..37

Part 2: Connect with Others...45

Chapter 5: Cherish Friendships.......................................47
Chapter 6: Communicate Needs & Boundaries.......55
Chapter 7: Speak Words of Life..65
Chapter 8: Seek Different Perspectives.......................75

Part 3: Embrace the Unknown 87

Chapter 9: Develop Inner Spirituality 89

Chapter 10: Find Purpose in Adversity 103

Chapter 11: Look for Opportunities to Grow 111

Chapter 12: Reflect on Your Progress 119

Conclusion 127

References 131

About the Author 135

Introduction

Peace and joy are not virtues we stumble upon, nor are we born with them. They are qualities we cultivate throughout our lives. We could all use more peace and joy. Stress, burnout, dissatisfaction, worry, and seemingly endless to-do lists often prevent us from living peaceful and joyful lives. However, the stressors and adversities of life are not obstacles to our peace and joy that we must remove; instead, they are circumstances during which we can nurture peace and happiness.

Just after my fiftieth birthday, I reflected on the life lessons I had learned and the things that helped me build a happier, more fulfilling life. I wrote these lessons on happiness as if I were sharing them with a friend suffering and needing extra hope. What resulted from my writing was a twelve-week journey toward lasting peace and joy. Each chapter is founded on research and life stories to illustrate the topic's scientific validity and demonstrate its practical use. Not all of these tips will resonate with you, which is okay! I hope that at least one or two will, and they will help you on your journey to inner peace and happiness in life.

In this book, you will explore three areas of life. Part 1 is about *accepting yourself*. This section will help you focus on the self-development and self-awareness necessary for increasing your peace and happiness. This is the start of the journey because it will inform every other part of the process, including the relationships you form, the activities you pursue, and the environments you create.

Part 2 is all about *connecting with others*. This section will give you the tools and wisdom to intentionally connect with people in your life. Healthy, thriving relationships are essential to living a happy life. The people we surround ourselves with and the words we speak play a huge role in cultivating more peace and joy.

After doing the internal work of self-acceptance and the external work of building healthy relationships, much of life is still unaccounted for, messy, and unknown—which can be scary. Part 3 focuses on *embracing the unknown*. When we stop and think about it, little is in our control. This section focuses on some of the unknowns and how we can be more okay with letting go of control so we can experience the fullness of life as it is happening.

I am a life-long educator who knows that adults learn by doing. You can read these words and get the lesson you yearned for; however, if you answer the reflection questions and do the activities, those lessons will sink deeper into your long-term memory, so you do not have to forget and relearn (like I have had to do so many times).

Here is how I recommend going through the book to get the most use out of it:

1. Read one chapter a week.

2. Answer the reflection questions.

3. Complete one of the activities listed or one of your own to implement the teaching into your life.

4. After one week of trying an activity or two, write a few paragraphs about what you did and how it went.

5. Move to the next chapter.

6. At the end of the book, pick one or two of your favorite chapters to continue to work on.

7. Share the book with a friend you believe might be helped by some of these lessons.

There are opportunities for joy and peace everywhere in your life. Through this journey, your eyes and mind will be open to the readily available self-acceptance around you. Spread kindness, be curious, and seek joy, my friends!

REFLECT

What do you hope to get out of this journey?

_____

_____

_____

_____

_____

_____

_____

_____

_____

_____

_____

_____

_____

_____

_____

_____

_____

_____

In what areas of your life are you seeking more peace and happiness?

_____

_____

_____

_____

_____

_____

_____

_____

_____

_____

_____

_____

_____

_____

_____

_____

_____

_____

_____

PART 1:

Accept Yourself

"*We have to dare to be ourselves,*
however frightening or strange
that self may prove to be."

— MAY SARTON

CHAPTER 1:
Practice Authenticity

"Authenticity is a collection of choices we must make daily. It's about the choice to show up and be real. The choice to be honest. The choice to let our true selves be seen."
— BRENE BROWN, *THE GIFTS OF IMPERFECTION*

Authenticity is a journey that takes time and effort to cultivate in your life—but living authentically leads to great happiness, fulfillment, and a stronger sense of self.

Living authentically means learning to be your true self in every situation. Deepak Chopra gives more information about what it means to be just that in his book *Living in the Light*:

"Your true self...is never wounded, cares nothing about criticism, sees everyone in the light of loving acceptance, and brings compassion and forgiveness to any situation" (Chopra and Platt-Finger).

Your true self is who you are when all the influences, criticism, and expectations of others fall away. It involves finding the values, beliefs, and preferences that best align with who you are and bring you peace. The hard part is digging deep to discover those beliefs, values, and preferences. In most homes, they are taught. That is a great starting point; however, as you age, step back and decide if what you have been taught resonates with *your* core values.

I have spent too much time wondering and worrying about what people think of me. I have learned through the years that this is a shallow and immature way to think. When striving to live authentically, you cannot worry about other people's thoughts. There will be many people who are critical of you. People in this group often have yet to find their own authenticity. They cannot understand your honesty, and they will be critical. That is hard to take at first.

It was not until I reached my forties that I let that go. You will not have authentic happiness if you constantly live to impress and appease others. Without knowing what people think, it can be tempting to make up a story and believe it as if it were fact. Humans waste much energy on these stories. I used to do this because I thought I could read people well. I have discovered that it is simply not true. It was just something I told myself so I could continue to believe the story I made up.

Living authentically has been a lengthy process for me. I grew up always wondering what people were thinking about me. I worried that what I wore, said, and did would not be acceptable. I met my husband in high school, and one of the things that impressed me the most was that he never worried about what others thought of him. That was a new concept to me as a teenage girl in a high school with a homogenous population: majority white, similar economic status, and most of the same religion. He lived authentically, and I had never met anyone like him. Frankly, I was jealous of his freedom. It seemed so refreshing. He deserves credit for starting me on my own truth journey!

When our kids were young, I made a conscious decision: I wanted them to be able to be themselves and live their truth. I planned to teach them what I knew and my perspective, but I would let them think for themselves and make their choices. That felt like a solid plan to build independent, authentically kind humans. However, giving up that control over their lives was not easy.

Later, as they grew into teens and young adults, they made choices that differed from my own judgment, so I had to stop, step back, and ask myself, "Are you willing to let them be their true selves?" I knew it was best for them, but it was tough not to try to control their choices. I would offer advice and give warnings but let them go with their guts on meaningful life decisions. I urged them to speak the truth and follow their instinct. I found that the more I understood and lived my truth, the more willing I was to let my children do the same. Our relationships strengthened, and they became more confident in their choices.

All these experiences have helped me to know myself so I can live vulnerably on the journey I am still on. While it is not easy, I have found that living my truth is the only way for me to have true inner peace and happiness.

Research has consistently shown that living authentically is positively associated with various aspects of well-being, including happiness. One study published in the *Journal of Personality and Social Psychology* found that individuals who acted following their true selves experienced greater well-being, self-esteem, and life satisfaction than those who did not. The study also found that individuals who reported feeling a greater sense of authenticity were more likely to engage in self-expression, contributing to their well-being.[1]

Another study published in the *Journal of Positive Psychology* found

---

1   Sheldon et al., 1996.

that individuals who lived more authentic lives reported more robust and less harmful emotions than those who lived less authentically. The study also found that living authentically was associated with greater resilience in adversity.[2] By letting go of what others think about us, we can find the freedom and space to be our true selves—and nothing is better for inner happiness and peace.

Humans have an innate need for belonging. This need supersedes the desire for authenticity in some stages of your life. This desire for belonging can cause us to withhold the truth and continue relationships with people who hurt us. This is done to strengthen your sense of belonging. However, once you feel a healthy sense of belonging with a particularly close group, you can start the growth journey of seeking an authentic life.

For some, love and belonging will always outweigh the need to be authentic. And for some, that is okay. My journey for authenticity has brought me much inner peace, but it took a long time for me to get there. Many people lean toward belonging rather than speaking their truth, and it is easy to judge them for that. I often struggle to understand why they continue relationships they do not enjoy or agree verbally with things they do not believe. I must remind myself that it is okay for others to lean toward belonging. I understand and empathize because while my quest to live authentically has brought me inner peace, it has changed my sense of belonging in certain circles. Some friendships have fallen away, but my intense need for authenticity outweighs my desire to belong where I cannot speak my truth.

The great author and professor Brené Brown said in her book Braving the Wilderness, "True belonging doesn't require you to change who you are; it requires you to be who you are." Brené Brown's research and writings about belonging have shed so much light on the work we can do to move more toward authenticity.

---

2   Wood, Linley, et al.

Living authentically is a profound journey that involves under-standing what truly matters to you. It requires deep soul-searching and rethinking everything. After a lifetime of listening to what others think, discovering your truth takes profound inner work. The work is more difficult when you have only listened to the outside world's view of who you are.

As I have moved toward my most authentic self, some friends and acquaintances have naturally left my life. It can be shocking initially if that happens, but please consider that those relationships may have existed on pretenses. The more you move toward your soul, the more shallow relationships diminish. However, loyal friendships with those who love you for who you are get stronger and more fulfilling.

There are countless influences in your daily life. People around you, social media, celebrities, and influencers tell us who to be and what to buy to become who we should be. To live more authentically, you must uncover what brings you joy, what makes you feel most like yourself, and what you value when there are no distractions. Learn from others, but be yourself. As you work toward living authentically, you can hold more space for others to do the same, leading to better relationships.

What are some things or activities that bring you joy? How can you incorporate them into your life more?

_____

_____

_____

_____

_____

_____

When and with whom do you feel most like yourself? How is what you value represented in those situations or with that person? What does that feel like?

_____

_____

_____

_____

_____

_____

_____

ACTIVITIES FOR WEEK 1:

1. Consider what you value most: belonging or authenticity. If you have an innate need to belong, consider if you are giving up part of who you are to belong to a group. Would that group accept you if you showed your true self? Are you truly happy when you stifle your authentic self to belong? Be curious about these questions this week, and write down your thoughts.

2. Meditation is a beautiful space for this inner work of practicing authenticity. If you are new to meditation, I recommend finding a face-to-face course in your

community. I started with an MBSR (Mindfulness-Based Stress Reduction) course offered by my local county behavioral health services. That course revealed how meditation is not about quieting your thoughts. It is about letting your thoughts come and go without judgment. It is about looking deep inside your soul and letting go of anything not serving you. Doing this lets you listen to your inner voice and understand yourself more deeply. Yoga is also a movement meditation that helps balance your mind, body, and soul. Plenty of meditation apps are available that provide guided meditation or meditation music. Try them all and see what sticks in your life. Perhaps you are already meditating. Congrats! That is fantastic. Is it time to try a new format or expand your meditation practice? You decide what works best for you right now.

Write about your experience doing these activities:

_____

_____

_____

_____

_____

_____

_____

_____

_____

CHAPTER 2:
Establish Core Character

"Do not judge others. Be your own judge,
and you will be truly happy."
— MAHATMA GANDHI

Understanding your values and how you present yourself to the world is the cornerstone of self-discovery and self-acceptance. It is about recognizing what truly matters and aligning your actions with those beliefs. After working to understand your authentic self, the outward expression of your inner values and beliefs becomes fundamentally important. How you show yourself to others is an integral part of your happiness.

Balance of self-presentation with self-awareness is critical. It is not about appearing flawless or trying to impress others. Instead, it is about sharing your values and perspectives clearly and straightfor-wardly. This approach helps you connect with others more deeply and promotes a sense of self-acceptance.

Understanding your own core values can help you be less

judgmental of others. When you know what matters most to *you*, it is easier to understand how other people have their own values, too. We all come from different backgrounds and experiences. When someone does something different from what you would do, instead of jumping to judge, think, "Hey, maybe that is important to them." It is like stepping into their shoes and realizing there is more than one way to see things. Plus, it is a good reminder that just like you want your values respected, you should do the same for others.

I was assigned drop-off duty when I taught elementary school at our local neighborhood school. This means I had to stand at the entrance to the school drop-off area and ensure cars pulled forward and waited to drop the kids off until they were safe.

This is a dreaded assignment for teachers. Parent drivers do crazy things, and repeatedly reminding them of the rules can be frustrating. A few times, I saw a car doing something I deemed foolish, and I would instantly feel angry and start yelling at the car. As the vehicle approached me, it was often a good friend or neighbor behind the wheel, and it stopped me in my tracks. I was forgiving and kinder when I saw the person in the car.

These experiences were excellent reminders that *humans* were in the cars with different experiences and concerns. When I did not see them as "carpool parents" but rather as individual people, I could be empathetic and caring. When confronted with an opportunity to judge someone by their appearance or their actions, I remind myself that the person is someone's child, parent, or friend, and I do not know what they are dealing with in life. They are human beings with feelings. It helps me to be curious and kind rather than judgmental.

As you come to know your true inner self and realize that you may be different than you thought, your mind opens to how other people may be different than you initially thought. As my perspective has broadened over the years, I realize I do not necessarily fit all the stereotypes I have placed upon myself. For instance, I have spent much of my life trying to fit into the "box" where I thought I belonged. After some deep soul-searching, I realized no one truly fits into a box. Everyone has unique thoughts, feelings, reactions, and experiences—and they vary. We may all have some similarities, but we are all beautifully different. This realization helped me start to question basic stereotypes.

Vast amounts of research have been done on stereotypes over the years. After years of research, social psychologist Susan Fiske presented the Stereotype Content Model. The model explains the human innate tendency to judge people by the groups we perceive them to be in. We tend to meet people, place them into a category, and then make judgments based on the group with which we associate them.

People form opinions and make judgments about individuals or groups based on their perceived level of two aspects: warmth and competence. Warmth has to do with how friendly, trustworthy, and well-intentioned someone seems. Competence involves how skilled, intelligent, and capable they appear. Combinations of warmth and competence generate distinct emotions of admiration, contempt, envy, and pity.[1]

Fiske's work also shows that the more you get to know different people, the more you discover who you are. Therefore, you are likelier to drop the stereotyping and see the person for their characteristics.

---

1   Fiske, 2018. Stereotype Content: Warmth and Competence Endure. Current Directions in Psychological Science, 27(2), 67-73. https://doi.org/10.1177/ 0963721417738825

An article regarding the Stereotype Content Model states:

> "Stereotypes can be oversimplified, biased pathways
> through which we place people and ideas into discrete
> categories. Our tendency to rely on stereotypes means
> we are quick to judge a book by its cover and arrive at
> conclusions that may not be warranted. Even if our
> stereotypes presuppose positive characteristics, they
> still blind us to complex personhood and reduce people
> to a single story that we come to understand as truth."[2]

It is human nature to make these snap judgments about people. However, as you understand your innate differences, you will realize how these judgments are inaccurate and only tell part of the story.

Have you ever been the victim of someone else's incorrect judgment? I have, and it feels unfair, confusing, and hurtful. Have you ever judged someone immediately to find out later that you were wrong? I have, and it has left me feeling ashamed. Both of these instances involved erroneous perceptions, and neither felt good.

These types of experiences have helped me to stop myself from passing judgment on someone before I know them. The more life experiences you have, the more you broaden your perspective. A broad perspective can help you see past stereotypes and learn about people before making snap judgments. The more you practice this, the more inner peace you will develop.

---

2   "Reference Guide: Stereotypes." The Decision Lab.

Whose qualities do you admire?

Identify people you admire—whether they are historical figures, friends, family members, or public figures. What qualities or characteristics do you admire in them? The values we look up to in others often reflect our inner values, offering insights into what we hold dear.

_____

_____

_____

_____

_____

_____

_____

_____

_____

_____

_____

_____

_____

_____

_____

_____

_____

What matters even when no one is watching?

Consider the decisions you make when there is no external pressure or judgment. What choices do you consistently lean toward? These decisions might showcase your authentic values and character as they are not influenced by societal norms or others' opinions.

_____

_____

_____

_____

_____

_____

_____

_____

_____

_____

_____

_____

_____

_____

_____

ACTIVITIES FOR WEEK 2:

1. Learn to understand your inner strengths. The free Values in Action (VIA) Character Strengths Survey is a beautiful place to do this.[3] The test organizes your strengths into an ordered list with descriptions. The premise is that you encompass all twenty-four defined strengths at various levels. By focusing your efforts on emphasizing your top five character strengths, you will find more happiness and satisfaction in your life. Take the survey and then act on your strengths. Find ways to focus on them in your everyday life.

2. Spend this week curious about the stories of strangers. Strike up a conversation when possible and learn more about them. Lead with kindness rather than judgment.

Write about your experience doing these activities:

_____

_____

_____

_____

_____

_____

3   viacharacter.org

CHAPTER 3:
Value Imperfections

"Stop trying to 'fix' yourself; you are NOT broken! You are perfectly imperfect and powerful beyond measure."

— STEVE MARIBOLI

Imperfection and adversity are a natural part of the human experience. Accepting this reality can improve mental health by reducing stress, increasing resilience, and promoting a positive outlook.

When I was young, I aimed for perfection in everything I did. That led to much anxiety. When perfection is your goal, you get anxious because you aim for something unattainable.

No one told me I had to be perfect. My parents did the best they could, and they never placed that burden on me. Somehow, I put it on myself.

Academics were always critical to me, and I aimed to excel. While dating my now husband, Eric, during my sophomore year of high school, I was constantly stressed about grades. He was not. He was a carefree senior with no concerns. I remember being upset after receiving a C+ on my report card; it was the first time I received less than a B.

He said, "Do you think you will remember this grade a year from now?"

I had never thought about the long-term or big picture regarding perfection. I only considered that moment and how it made me feel. I thought about his statement and realized that my C+ would not affect my long-term goals. That was the beginning of a perception switch for me. I started not to worry so much about grades and focus more on what I was learning.

Raising children is an excellent exercise in realizing your imperfections. Even the parents who seem to have figured it all out screw up. I have known amazing parents who have raised disengaged children, and I have known parents who are complete amateurs who have raised obedient children. From my perspective, it all seems somewhat unpredictable.

I was never a perfect parent. I had to focus on loving my kids with all my heart and apologizing when I screwed up. In turn, I did not expect perfection from them. I expected them to live a life that brought them inner peace and happiness. It helped me a ton to focus on those things. The weight of knowing that my imperfections could impact their lives was heavy. I had to go easy on myself and focus on the big picture: loving my kids and helping them turn mistakes into lessons. Concentrating on that big picture allowed me to look past inadequacies.

I have done a complete one-eighty since my teenage years. I now embrace imperfection. I love people for who they are and for their unique journeys. I constantly make mistakes, say and do dumb or hurtful things without thinking, and misjudge others. All I can do is work to recognize when I do wrong and apologize. I have had harrowing experiences where I later realized my fault. In those times, it is hard to swallow your pride and apologize to anyone you hurt. Nevertheless, it is always worth it when you do. It can mend relationships and help you grow.

Research has shown that individuals with a greater acceptance of life's imperfections have better mental health outcomes. For example, a study published in the *Journal of Social and Clinical Psychology* found that acceptance of imperfection was associated with lower levels of anxiety and depression. The study also found that individuals with greater acceptance of their flaws had higher life satisfaction levels.[1] Studies have also shown that individuals who are more accepting of their imperfections can better form meaningful relationships with others. A study published in the *Journal of Personality and Social Psychology* found that more self-compassionate individuals are likely to form close friendships and romantic relationships.[2]

Life is **messy, unpredictable**, and **beautiful** simultaneously. Embrace all three of those adjectives in your life. Expecting things to be perfect will only lead to disappointment. Nothing will throw you off when you embrace disorder as a natural part of everyday life. Life is beautiful because our growth lies in messiness and unpredictability.

By being flexible and living in service of your deepest values instead of being narrowly focused on achieving happiness, you end up experiencing more frequent joy and meaning in life and less distress; you end up with greater vitality and degrees of freedom for how to live each moment.

Life is not perfect; it is messy, unpredictable, and beautiful. The sooner you realize that, the sooner you will start to let your expectations of yourself and others be more flexible. As that happens, you learn to hold the messiness, recognizing the growth of embracing imperfection.

---

1   Kashdan & Rottenberg, 2010.
2   Neff & Beretvas, 2013.

What have your mistakes taught you?

Reflect on times when things did not go as planned or when you made what you might consider a mistake. What did you learn from those situations? Often, our imperfections are powerful teachers, showing us new paths and perspectives we would not have discovered otherwise.

_____

_____

_____

_____

_____

_____

_____

_____

_____

_____

_____

_____

_____

_____

_____

How have your imperfections shaped your growth?

Consider how your imperfections have contributed to your personal growth and development. Have they pushed you to develop new skills and become more resilient or empathetic? Imperfections can be catalysts for positive change.

_____

_____

_____

_____

_____

_____

What would you say to a friend in the same situation?

Imagine a friend confiding in you about their imperfections or mistakes. What advice and support would you offer them? Sometimes, giving ourselves the same kindness and understanding we give to others can help us embrace our imperfections with compassion.

_____

_____

_____

_____

_____

_____

_____

ACTIVITIES FOR WEEK 3:

1. Forgive yourself for your shortcomings. Embrace the idea that you are not perfect and no one should expect you to be. Throughout the week, when you realize a mistake, stop and say to yourself, "I love and respect myself. I do not need to be perfect; I must be kind to myself and others."

2. Focus on your strengths. Go back to your top five strengths from the VIA Character Strengths. Write them somewhere that you will see daily. Focus on them instead of perfection.

Write about your experience doing these activities:

_____

_____

_____

_____

_____

_____

_____

_____

CHAPTER 4:
Get Curious

"Be curious. Not judgmental."
—WALT WHITMAN

Living with non-judgmental curiosity helps you learn more about other people's perspectives. Real growth comes as you seek knowledge and understanding through curiosity. You will learn more about yourself when seeking understanding about others.

I started to learn about the benefits of curiosity during meditation practice. The goal of meditation is not to stop your thoughts; it is to notice the thoughts that pass through your mind and not judge them. It is about being curious about them. When you learn to do this with your thoughts, it translates to your experiences in life. It encourages you not to react to things that happen with snap judgments but instead pause, wonder, and be curious about what is happening. That might sound simple, but it is radical in helping you handle life experiences and relationships in a way that inspires inner peace and happiness.

When you make mistakes, try to be curious about them. When you meet someone with a different lifestyle or belief system, try to be curious about what makes them tick. If you think about it, curiosity is synonymous with open-mindedness. To be curious about others means you are interested in what led them to where they are or attentive to what they believe or do. Curious means "eager to know or learn something."

Being curious is a great way to go about life. Using curiosity rather than judgment is like flipping a switch in your brain. When you are curious, you are open to new ideas and perspectives. You are not quick to label things or people. This mindset can boost your peace and happiness game. Why? Because curiosity helps you see the world as a learning playground rather than a judgment arena.

When you are curious, you are less stressed about right or wrong. You are like a detective trying to understand things. This takes the pressure off, and less pressure usually means more peace.

Curiosity encourages you to ask questions, often leading to deeper connections and a better understanding of people around you. Strong connections add to your inner happiness.

Todd Kashdan, an American psychologist and director of the Well-Being Laboratory at George Mason University, said curiosity leads to a multitude of life-fulfilling benefits, including managing anxiety, reducing defensive reactions when threatened, encouraging innovation, and serving as a source of resilience when exposed to adverse life events and stressors.

When problems arise, take an inquisitive approach; it will help you see things from a less critical, big-picture standpoint, which helps resolve issues.

When something happens, you can choose if and how to react. Before you react, if you take a second to pause and be curious about what happened, it can help you respond in a more calm and non-judgmental manner. Be curious about your initial reactions.

It also helps you abandon the idea that you are always right. When you always think you know the correct answer, you can become critical of others who do not feel like you do. However, when you are curious about other peoples' points of view, it helps you be more open-minded and realize that your answers are not always suitable for everyone.

A few phrases to use in conversations to avoid judgment include, "Tell me more about that..." and "I am curious why you think..." Whenever you feel an instant need to judge or jump to conclusions about something someone has said or done, pause and ask one of these questions. It will help you understand the person and their motives better.

What are you taking for granted?

Reflect on aspects of your daily life that you might be overlooking or taking for granted. What if you approached them with fresh curiosity? This shift can help you find wonder in the ordinary and boost your inner peace.

_____

_____

_____

_____

_____

_____

_____

_____

How can you listen with genuine interest?

Consider how you engage in conversation. Are you truly curious about what others are saying or just waiting for your turn to speak? Challenge yourself to listen genuinely, asking questions to understand others' perspectives deeply.

_____

_____

_____

_____

_____

_____

_____

_____

_____

_____

_____

_____

_____

What can you explore outside your comfort zone?

Think about something you have always been curious about but have yet to explore. It could be a hobby, a new topic, or a different social circle. Stepping out of your comfort zone with an open mind can lead to exciting discoveries and enriched relationships.

_____

_____

_____

_____

_____

_____

_____

_____

_____

_____

_____

_____

_____

_____

_____

ACTIVITIES FOR WEEK 4:

1. Take a few minutes each day to engage in mindful observation. Choose an object, a scene, or even a person, and observe it with genuine curiosity. Notice the details you might usually overlook—colors, textures, shapes. As you do this, try to suspend any judgments or assumptions that come up. This practice can train your mind to be present, curious, and non-judgmental.

2. During your conversations with others, purposefully take on the role of being curious rather than judgmental. When someone shares an opinion or perspective that differs from your own, instead of immediately disagreeing or forming a judgment, say things like, "Tell me more about that," or "Help me understand that better." This exercise can help you develop empathy and broaden your perspective.

Write about your experience doing these activities:

_____

_____

_____

_____

_____

_____

PART 2:
Connect with Others

"Ye live not for yourselves; ye cannot live for yourselves; a thousand fibers connect you with your fellowmen, and along those fibers, as along sympathetic threads, run your actions as causes and return to you as effects."

—HENRY MELVILL

CHAPTER 5:
Cherish Friendships

"Friendship is unnecessary, like philosophy, like art... It has no survival value; rather, it is one of those things which give value to survival."

—C.S. LEWIS, *THE FOUR LOVES*

True friendship is a bond that goes beyond just enjoying the company or having shared interests. It involves accepting and loving someone for who they are, flaws and all, and supporting them in their journey.

About twenty years ago, a neighbor of mine asked if I would be interested in walking with her in the mornings for exercise. I agreed, and that was the beginning of our beautiful relationship. Our twenty years of friendship have included babysitting swaps, family vacations together, job loss, divorce, faith changes, and a slew of other desirable and not-so-desirable experiences. We are not who we were when we started our journey together. We have been stretched, pushed, moved, and hurt through various life experiences. We have been through times when we saw each other every day and times when we barely spoke for months. Through it all, our friendship has expanded and grown into something priceless. We started out loving each other for our similarities and grew into admiring each other for our differences. I have learned more from listening to her perspective than I ever could have learned from my own.

COVID-19 was a tremendous human personality trait experiment. During quarantine, it was easy to tell who was an introvert and an extrovert. Some of my family members lost their minds when they had to stay home and not interact with others. I had one daughter who would hop in her car and drive for hours, talking on the phone to friends. She could not stand being cooped up. (She is an extrovert, if that wasn't clear). On the other hand, I was in heaven, staying home with no obligations to go anywhere or interact with anyone other than my family. I was in my comfort zone with no reason to leave it. That was my first realization that I am an introvert.

When I discovered that about myself (I always knew it but was in denial for some reason), I started to be kinder to myself. I realized that my whole life, I have valued and cherished a small number of unique relationships as opposed to a million friends. That works for me! The friends who love me understand that I do not need to see them daily, do not desire to attend parties (ask my friends how I feel about attending baby or bridal showers, too. So painful for me!), and do not want to be the center of attention. I am an excellent listener, and I love supporting a friend in need. That sounds like a true introvert to me!

As a side note, I also realized that I had been drawn to extroverts my entire life. Most of my friends throughout the years have been extroverted, along with most of my immediate family members. It makes sense why I sometimes need a moment to be alone and gather my thoughts. I always felt selfish for needing that, but now I know it is just part of who I am.

True friendships come in many ways. Sometimes, it is a family member, a lifelong friend, a new acquaintance, or a coworker. Learn to recognize true friendships as the people you do not have to pretend with, the ones who love you for who you are, burdens and all. A great litmus test for true friendship is a good old-fashioned life challenge.

When you have experienced hard times or been down, who is there for you no matter what? Those are your true friends. If you have friends who are constantly your critics, you may want to look for new ones. True friends will build you up, support you, and be honest with you. Look for friends who do these things. And then, in turn, be that kind of friend to others. Be the person who supports, cries with, and cheers on your friends. Leave jealousy and judgment, comparison, and complaints behind, and be a devoted friend to others.

Perhaps you have many friends who fall into this category. Good for you! Take a step back and ensure *you* are *also* being a good friend. Cherish those relationships and do everything you can to support and love those friends.

Perhaps you have yet to make friends who fall into this category. That is okay, too. Start taking applications now, figuratively speaking. Start looking for those you admire and be a good friend to them. If they are authentic and kind, they will reciprocate.

Research has shown that true friendship has positive effects and can help individuals cope with stress and adversity. One study published in *Personal Relationships* found that close friendships were associated with greater life satisfaction and well-being. The study also found that friendship quality was more important than the number of friends in terms of well-being outcomes.[1]

The *Journal of Social Science & Medicine* states that social support from friends is associated with lower stress levels and better mental health outcomes. The study found that having friends who provide

---

1   Demir et al., 2011.

emotional and instrumental support helps individuals cope with stressors more effectively.[2]

Another study published in the *Journal of Personality and Social Psychology* found that having supportive friends could help individuals recover from negative experiences more quickly. The study found that individuals with a solid social support network were more resilient in the face of adversity and had better mental health outcomes.[3]

The research suggests that true friendship involves accepting and supporting individuals in their journey. Loyal friends provide emotional and instrumental support, and they can help individuals cope with stress and adversity more effectively. By cultivating true friendships, you can experience greater well-being and resilience.

Finding inner peace through friendships will be different for everyone, and rightfully so. Everyone has different personality traits and needs. Your need for friendships will also ebb and flow naturally with varying phases of life. During the years when I stayed home raising little kids all day, I was exhausted. I needed time away from my everyday life to be with my friends, whether it was a quick trip for ice cream on a weeknight or a getaway for a weekend; those times were essential to my inner peace. Now that I am older and have fewer responsibilities for raising my children, I cherish weekly lunches with friends to chat and catch up. We do not get together much, but our friendships are still as strong as ever.

Seek the type of friendships that fill your cup and bring you inner peace through your distinct phases of life. Furthermore, be the kind of friend who gives that friendship in return. If you do this, your friendships will be cherished and bring more happiness into your life than you could ever imagine.

---

2   Kawachi and Berkman, 2001.

3   Gable et al., 2004.

Why do you value your closest friends?

Reflect on the specific qualities and experiences that make your closest friendships meaningful. Consider how these friendships have supported you in various aspects of your life.

_____

_____

_____

_____

_____

_____

_____

_____

_____

_____

_____

_____

_____

_____

_____

_____

_____

_____

How can you actively cultivate and nurture true friendships?
Think about the steps you can take to strengthen and build new friendships. Consider how you can be more attentive, supportive, and understanding in your interactions. Reflect on the role you play in maintaining healthy friendships.

_____

_____

_____

_____

_____

_____

_____

_____

_____

_____

_____

_____

_____

_____

_____

_____

ACTIVITIES FOR WEEK 5:

1. Consider what type of friend you are. Write down your strengths and weaknesses as a friend and set goals to improve your ability to love and support the people you cherish.

2. Describe the characteristics of a good friend. Write them down and strive to be the type of friend who builds others up.

Write about your experience doing these activities:

_____

_____

_____

_____

_____

_____

_____

_____

_____

_____

CHAPTER 6:
Communicate Needs & Boundaries

"Incredible change happens in your life when you decide to take control of what you do have power over instead of craving control over what you don't."
—STEVE MARABOLI

You cannot control the actions, beliefs, or behaviors of others. You can only control your own actions and reactions to the world around you. Understanding this concept can lead to self-improvement and help you focus on personal growth rather than trying to change others.

When my kids were all in their teenage years, I had my daughter paint me a sign for my house with these words: *"You cannot change other people; you can only change yourself."* This was a running theme in my advice as they navigated those difficult years. Your power lies not in trying to change others but in improving yourself. It's highly influential. It can help you focus on what you can do to help relationships. When someone is treating you poorly, you can tell them how it makes you feel, and if they do not care, your power lies in walking away. I have had many experiences where things were not going how I thought they should be in a relationship, personally or professionally. By remembering where my power lies, I took a step back and considered how my actions affect things and what I could do differently.

In addition to the words on the sign in my house, I often remind myself to "focus on what I can control and let the rest go." As an adult, I have learned that many things in life are out of my control. I can spend my days stewing about that, and it will not change a thing. Alternatively, I can focus on what I can control: my reaction, emotion, and response. Those things are my responsibility; I am calmer and more peaceful if I concentrate on them.

One of the hardest things I have worked to do is not worry about unkind, cruel, and untrue things others say about me. It can be so tricky. I naturally want to clarify things and ensure people do not believe these untrue words. As I considered the best way to do this, I realized that my response was the only part I could control. I have to live so that if people know me, they will not believe incorrect gossip about me. That is my responsibility. Be kind, treat others well, and build relationships so cruel words from others will not affect you.

Part of accepting what you cannot change is learning to set healthy boundaries in your relationships. If you have someone who constantly criticizes you, oozes negativity, or speaks poorly of you to others, you can't always change their behavior, but you can set a healthy boundary. This is not done to punish the other person. It is a way to improve your inner peace and help you move forward on a healthier path. A boundary may include something as small as not discussing specific topics with a person or as extreme as not being around the person at all. Sometimes, it is about saying "no" to someone who takes advantage of your time or maybe just being more honest about not wanting to commit to specific activities. Find the right balance, communicate your boundary, and then stick to it for as long as necessary for your mental health. The boundary may change when you feel ready, but that should be your decision. Honestly and openly setting boundaries does not come easy, and there are often consequences; however, the peace from doing this generally outweighs the consequences.

Surround yourself with people who build you up, support your boundaries, and help you see the good in life. Use criticism to improve where you can, but do not allow others' negative words about you to bring you down. Remember that your control lies in your reactions and your emotions.

Research in psychology supports this concept. For example, a study published in the *Journal of Personality and Social Psychology* found that people who had an internal locus of control, or a belief that they had control over their own lives, tended to be more successful and have better mental health outcomes than those with an external locus of control.[1]

Additionally, a literature review on behavior-change interventions found that successful interventions often focus on providing patients with tools to cope with external factors rather than attempting to change the external factors themselves.[2] This supports the idea that focusing on personal change rather than trying to change others can lead to more successful outcomes.

Understanding that you cannot change others and can only change yourself leads to healthier relationships. Instead of changing others to fit your expectations, you can focus on accepting them for who they are and communicating your needs and boundaries.

---

1   Rotter, 1966.
2   Michie et al., 2011.

What aspects of your life are within your control, and which are beyond?

Begin by identifying the areas of your life where you have influence and control. Reflect on how to allocate your time, energy, and resources more effectively by concentrating on these aspects. Accepting the limits of power is a fundamental step in setting healthy boundaries.

_____

_____

_____

_____

_____

_____

_____

_____

_____

_____

_____

_____

_____

_____

_____

What are the signs that indicate you need to set boundaries in specific relationships or situations?

Reflect on past experiences where you felt overwhelmed, stressed, or drained due to over-commitment or lack of boundaries. Consider the warning signs and emotional cues that indicate the need for boundaries in specific contexts. Recognize that setting boundaries is a proactive act of self-care.

How can I communicate my boundaries assertively and respectfully?

Explore strategies for effectively communicating your boundaries to others. Reflect on ways to express your needs and limits clearly and respectfully, emphasizing your commitment to maintaining healthy relationships and personal well-being. Consider how you can reinforce these boundaries consistently over time.

_____

_____

_____

_____

_____

_____

_____

_____

_____

_____

_____

_____

_____

_____

_____

ACTIVITIES FOR WEEK 6:

1. Dedicate time to self-reflection this week. Set aside a few minutes daily to contemplate your thoughts, emotions, and experiences. Reflect on situations where you felt in control and situations where you struggled with boundaries. Ask yourself what you can learn from these experiences and how you can apply those lessons.

2. Set a few clear goals and priorities for your life. Define what you want to achieve and what truly matters to you. This activity helps you identify where you should invest your time and energy, aligning with what you can control. Regularly review and adjust your goals to remain relevant to your evolving needs.

3. Incorporate mindfulness and relaxation techniques into your daily routine this week. Deep breathing exercises, progressive muscle relaxation, or short mindfulness sessions contribute to increased self-awareness and boundary-setting.

Write about your experience doing these activities:

_____

_____

_____

_____

_____

_____

_____

_____

_____

_____

_____

_____

_____

_____

_____

_____

_____

_____

_____

_____

_____

_____

_____

_____

CHAPTER 7:
Speak Words of Life

"Acceptance is simply love in practice. When you love, you accept; when you lack love, you judge."
—ABHIJIT NASKAR

Shifting your thoughts and words toward life and unity, rather than division and tearing people down, is crucial to finding inner peace. Two strategies for doing this are avoiding gossip and respecting diverse ways of thinking.

I have known gossipers and have been one at times. It can be a natural reaction to participate in gossip. The key is to realize when you are participating in it and stop the behavior. Changing the trajectory of relationships habitually based on tearing others down with gossip can be challenging. When I am placed in a situation where others gossip, I must stop myself from adding to the conversation. I also try to see things from other perspectives. While challenging to do with kindness, it is worth the effort, as you will find more life satisfaction when you focus on fixing your faults rather than analyzing others.

Although gossip can be entertaining and provide a sense of community, it can harm individuals and relationships. Research has shown that gossip can harm happiness in several ways. It can lead to guilt, shame, and embarrassment, damaging self-esteem and social relationships. Additionally, gossiping can create a hostile social environment and perpetuate harmful stereotypes and biases. Also, being the target of gossip can lead to feelings of betrayal, mistrust, and isolation.

While gossip serves some social functions, be mindful of the potential harm it can cause individuals and relationships. By doing so, you can work to create more positive and supportive social environments.

Unfortunately, gossip is very prevalent in society. Whether among family members, a group of friends, or a team of coworkers, we are all prone to talking about others when they are absent.

Venting is not gossip. Venting is "to give free expression to a strong emotion." Gossip is spread maliciously while venting relieves pent-up frustration. Venting can be a healthy way to express yourself. If a person has made you upset or angry, venting can help you release the emotions. It allows you to communicate your feelings instead of holding them in. If you vent with the right people, you can gain insight from their perspective on the situation. Venting improves your thinking and creates strong relationships with the listener.

We all have times when challenging things occur involving other people in our lives. In these circumstances, venting is appropriate. Venting with a trusted friend can help you to express your frustrations productively. Gossip, however, has a different motive. The motive of gossip is to destroy someone's reputation. It is done to push someone down and build yourself up.

I have acquaintances who have experienced trauma and hurt from others. They will often talk together about experiences and frustrations regarding these relationships. They do this to support each other and help each other heal and move on. This is not gossip. This is venting. This can be a form of therapy.

Embracing diverse perspectives can help you avoid gossip and speak "words of life." It reflects a broader societal shift toward promoting harmony and cooperation. So often, we focus on our thoughts and beliefs and see different ways of thinking as threats. It is vital to embrace other perspectives and approach them with tolerance and empathy. This can lead to a more mature understanding of our belief systems and unity in our relationships.

In Jonathan Haidt's *The Coddling of the American Mind*, he writes, "Morality binds and blinds. This is not just something that happens to people on the other side. We all get sucked into tribal moral communities. We circle around sacred values and then share post hoc arguments about why we are so right and they are so wrong. We think the other side is blind to truth, reason, science, and common sense, but in fact, everyone goes blind when talking about their sacred objects."

This way of thinking is prevalent in our world today. As our political parties, social groups, and religions go to extremes, we see more and more dichotomous thinking. When you are stuck in an extreme mindset, seeing things from another person's perspective is difficult. The more you focus on your own perceptions, the more extreme your thinking becomes. When we converse with people who think differently from us with curiosity and respect for them, we can grow our perspective and understand others better. We do not have to agree, but we *must* respect diverse ways of thinking and living to improve our world and our happiness and inner peace. Thinking your beliefs are the only correct and relevant ones is immature. Respecting others and letting them live and believe the way they feel is right for them is a sign of maturity.

We all have blind spots. No one is correct one hundred percent of the time. Realizing that will help you accept that life is complex and that many other beautiful shades exist besides black and white.

Scholarly research highlights the significance of shifting our thoughts and words toward life and unity. Drawing from principles of positive psychology, you can foster a more harmonious and inclusive society and contribute to a culture of understanding, empathy, and cooperation, ultimately working toward a better future for all.

Emphasizing positive aspects through your words and actions can foster unity and mutual support, as highlighted in Barbara L. Fredrickson's "The Broaden-and-Build Theory of Positive Emotions."[1] Fredrickson's theory suggests that positive emotions broaden an individual's mindset, making them more open to diverse perspectives and fostering social bonds. Positive language and thoughts can be pivotal in creating a supportive environment within individual and collective contexts.

Martin Seligman, one of the fathers of positive psychology, has provided insights into how focusing on positive attributes can significantly enhance life satisfaction and promote a more optimistic perspective.[2] Another study by Lyubomirsky et al. delves into the connection between positive emotions and personal success.[3] Their research reveals that focusing on positive words and actions contributes to individual well-being and enhances one's ability to attain personal and professional achievements.

Learn to recognize gossip as hurtful and work to avoid it. Listen to other's perspectives and realize that it's okay for them to see things differently. Doing this will help you be more positive and open-minded, creating more happiness and inner peace.

---

1   Philosophical Transactions of the Royal Society B, 2004.
2   American Psychologist, 2000.
3   "The Benefits of Frequent Positive Affect: Does Happiness Lead to Success?" Psychological Bulletin, 2005.

How do your words and thoughts impact the people around you?

Reflect on past interactions, recognize instances where negativity or divisiveness may have hindered unity, and then contrast them with moments of positivity and support that fostered a sense of togetherness.

_____

_____

_____

_____

_____

_____

_____

_____

_____

_____

_____

_____

_____

_____

_____

_____

_____

How can you actively practice empathy and constructive communication?

Think about how you can engage in constructive conversations that build bridges rather than walls in your relationships and within broader society.

_____

_____

_____

_____

_____

_____

_____

_____

_____

_____

_____

_____

_____

_____

_____

ACTIVITIES FOR WEEK 7:

1. Stop and listen the next time you are in an argument or heated discussion. Put more energy into understanding the other person's point of view than you put into proving you are right.

2. For one day, set a goal to talk about people only if they are in the room with you.

3. When tempted by gossip, be curious about what insecurities are causing you to find joy in tearing down someone else.

Write about your experience doing these activities:

_____

_____

_____

_____

_____

_____

_____

_____

_____

CHAPTER 8:
Seek Different Perspectives

"Our ability to reach unity in diversity
will be the beauty and the test of our civilization."
—MAHATMA GANDHI

Being exposed only to people who share your ideas, beliefs, and perspectives can limit your personal growth and development. Diversity of thought and experiences is necessary for personal growth.

More than thirty years ago, I met my husband. We could not be more different in every way possible. We often laugh at how we pick the opposite of each other in most choices. His perspective on life has been the most valuable thing to my growth. His thoughts on politics, religion, raising kids, and other crucial topics differ significantly from mine. Nevertheless, they have helped me to learn more about myself and to stretch my perspective.

It was not until I had a friend who is gay that I started to understand the perspectives of LGBTQ+ people. It was not until I started listening to someone with differing political values that I saw the wisdom in their thinking. It was not until I truly listened to a friend with a mental illness that I started empathizing with those who suffer. I learned to see other perspectives when I sat with an atheist and listened to their beliefs.

It is hard for me to admit that I had never taken the time to understand the perspective of other cultures and races. I was in my forties when I had a horrible realization. It was when my home state started recognizing Juneteenth as a holiday, and I wanted to know more about what it represented. A quick internet search and a bit of other research made me realize that July 4, the holiday I have always loved and revered because of the patriotism my military family taught me, was not a day of independence for all Americans. The public school system, the same one that taught me about Martin Luther King Jr., Rosa Parks, and Harriet Tubman, failed to help me see another perspective. The enslaved people were not freed on July 4, 1776. That is primarily a white American Independence Day, and most of my white American friends and I had no idea. That is shameful, and it is a result of only seeing things from my white, patriotic viewpoint.

You never grow when you surround yourself with people who think like you. Read that again. It is one of the most vital things I have ever learned. Consider your chosen relationships—your marriage and your friendships. Do you pick people who think like you? Do you tend to leave relationships with people who disagree with your perspective or live different lifestyles from you?

Lean into relationships that will open your mind and help you see the world from other viewpoints. You will only agree with some, and that is the point. Mature people can be friends with others with whom they disagree. So often, we push away from those who think differently. Republicans abhor Democrats; Democrats criticize Republican thinking. God-fearing people stay away from atheists. How will we unite to make a better world if we continue that path?

The social psychologist and author Jonathan Haidt says this better than I can in many of his books. If you want to learn more about this concept, I urge you to read his books. From *The Happiness Hypothesis* to his essay "The Coddling of the American Mind," he describes how we can learn to understand others and work together for good. One of my favorite quotes from his writings is below:

"An important dictum of cultural psychology is that each culture develops expertise in some aspects of human existence, but no culture can be expert in all aspects… Therefore, a good place to look for wisdom is where you least expect to find it: in the minds of your opponents. You already know the ideas common on your own side. If you can take off the blinders of the myth of pure evil, you might see some good ideas for the first time."

It is also important to point out that we fear what we do not understand. To understand someone better, you must listen.

Another important aspect of seeking out diverse perspectives is to avoid black-and-white thinking. Any method of thinking that involves "I am always right, and you are always wrong" will lead to conditional love, poor relationships, and a lack of inner peace. Black-and-white thinking, or dichotomous thinking, is a cognitive distortion involving perceiving situations and experiences in all-or-nothing terms without recognizing nuances or gray areas. This thinking can lead to judgment and self-righteousness, creating rigid and inflexible beliefs about yourself and others.

Dichotomous thinking leads to self-righteousness and a sense of moral superiority. A study published in the *Journal of Personality and Social Psychology* found that individuals who engaged in black-and-white thinking were more likely to endorse moral absolutes and to view themselves as more virtuous than others.[1] It creates rigid and inflexible beliefs about yourself and others. This thinking can also lead to adverse outcomes, such as anxiety, depression, interpersonal

---

1   Malka et al., 2010.

conflict, and prejudice.

Living in a community that mirrors yourself can lead to this dangerous thinking. Sometimes, strict religious practices will lead here also. It keeps you from seeing the world as complex and full of all the beautiful shades and colors that fall in between. It mostly comes from a need for more understanding. The more you experience life, the more you realize it is complex and messy sometimes.

Some great advice is never to assume that your thinking is always correct. Always second-guess your rightness. This little exercise can help you check yourself and be more open to other perspectives.

Dichotomous or black-and-white thinking is dangerous. It is often based on some idea of attainable perfection. It gives you only two alternatives: perfection and imperfection. When you believe these are the only two ways to live, you put too much pressure on yourself and too much pressure on others to enjoy fulfilling relationships.

I have known people who follow this line of thinking. Things go okay for them at first, but eventually, others around them cannot take the nonstop judgment. Over the years, honest and loving people started to fall out of their lives, leaving only relationships with other binary thinkers. This can be dangerous because, as a group, they start to validate each other as they discuss their dichotomous delusions. This leads to even more black-and-white, self-righteous beliefs that exclude everyone who might have a chance of helping them broaden their perspective and find inner peace. It is a horrible cycle to watch, especially for those who can see it for what it is: an unhealthy slope that leads to isolation, sadness, and pain.

Please know that if you are stuck in a trap of judging others for their righteousness based on your standards, you must stop. You will never find true happiness in such deception. Your love will be conditional on people living up to your expectations, which are impossible to attain. It is difficult to consider the beautiful relationships I would never have developed if I expected everyone to live, believe, and act like me. I would miss out on lovely relationships and the inner strength and wisdom I have gained from others.

I do not believe that religions teach this as doctrine. It is a human interpretation of righteousness. I also recognize that some mental illnesses can cause extreme ideas. However, no matter the origin, I cannot believe it will ever lead to inner peace and happiness.

A myriad of research has demonstrated the impact of diversity on individual growth. For instance, a study published in the Journal of Personality and Social Psychology found that individuals exposed to diverse perspectives exhibited greater creativity and innovation than those exposed to homogeneous (similar) views.[2] The study suggested that exposure to diverse perspectives can lead to more complex cognitive structures and the ability to generate more diverse ideas.

Levine and Moreland's observation is consistent with findings from other studies. For instance, a meta-analysis conducted by Richard et al. reviewed the literature on cultural intelligence and found that individuals with higher levels of cultural diversity exposure tend to be more creative and adaptive in cross-cultural settings.[3]

Beyond individual creativity, research has consistently shown that diversity can profoundly impact organizations and societies. A study by Scott Page in "The Difference: How the Power of Diversity Creates Better Groups, Firms, Schools, and Societies" emphasizes that diverse teams tend to outperform homogeneous ones in problem-solving and decision-making tasks.[4] This is because diverse teams bring various perspectives and approaches, leading to more effective and innovative solutions.

A wealth of research supports the idea that diversity significantly enhances creativity, innovation, problem-solving abilities,

---

2   Levine & Moreland, 1994.
3   "Cultural Intelligence: A Review, Reflections, and Recommendations for Future Research," International Journal of Intercultural Relations, 2009.
4   Princeton et al., 2007.

decision-making effectiveness, and personal growth. These benefits apply to individuals and profoundly impact organizations and societies, making diversity a critical factor in personal and professional development.

Find ways to expand your viewpoint. We are all on different journeys in life. We have individual experiences, thoughts, and reactions. Our job is to work on our journey and let others do the same. There is no need to judge if you live your journey "correctly." No one has the right to do that.

Make friends with those different from you; listen to those you do not understand. This will open your mind, heal your heart, and make you happier

How diverse are your sources of information and influence?
Reflect on the books, websites, media, and people that shape your worldview. Are they diverse in terms of culture, background, and perspective? Consider expanding your sources to include a broader range of voices and viewpoints.

What biases or preconceived notions might be influencing your judgments?

Take a critical look at your own biases and prejudices. Reflect on how these biases might impact your ability to embrace diverse perspectives. Challenge yourself to confront and address these biases to create a more inclusive mindset.

_____

_____

_____

_____

_____

_____

_____

_____

_____

_____

_____

_____

_____

_____

_____

_____

_____

Are you actively seeking conversations and experiences that expose you to different viewpoints?

Consider your social interactions and the conversations you engage in regularly. Are you actively seeking out opportunities to engage with people from diverse backgrounds and with differing opinions? Reflect on how you can intentionally create spaces for these interactions to occur.

_____

_____

_____

_____

_____

_____

_____

_____

_____

_____

_____

_____

_____

_____

_____

ACTIVITY FOR WEEK 8:

1. Find someone you know with a different perspective on life than yours and start conversing with them more on subjects that make you uncomfortable.

   Examples:

   - Find someone whose sexual preference differs from your own and respectfully listen to their experiences.

   - Find someone whose political views differ from yours and listen with respectful curiosity rather than judgment.

   - Find someone with different religious or spiritual beliefs, listen, and learn about their perspective. Do not judge. Only be curious.

2. Read a book from an author whose beliefs differ from yours. Set a goal to remain non-judgmental as you read and try to understand their perspective.

Write about your experience doing these activities:

_____

_____

_____

_____

_____

_____

_____

_____

_____

_____

_____

_____

_____

_____

_____

_____

_____

_____

_____

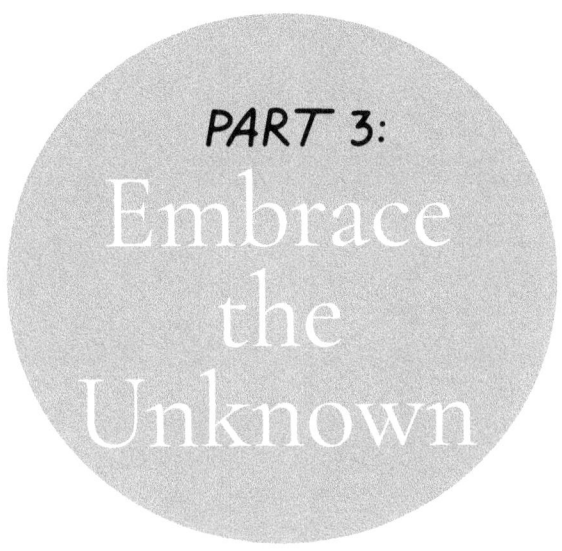

PART 3:
Embrace
the
Unknown

"*Relinquish your attachment to the known, step into the unknown,*
and you will step into the field of all possibilities."

— **DEEPAK CHOPRA**

CHAPTER 9:
Develop Inner Spirituality

*"All mature spirituality, in one sense or another,
is about letting go and unlearning."*
— **RICHARD ROHR, BREATHING UNDER WATER**

Working to understand your spirituality leads to inner peace. A simple internet search for the definition of spirituality will lead you to several options. The one I have heard that resonates most with me is "a sense of connection to something larger than yourself." The reason I like that definition is because it is so inclusive. It includes feeling connected to God, another higher power, the earth, nature, humanity, etc.

As a parent, I always relied on inspiration and obedience to God to help my children. I felt that if I did everything God asked me to do, I would be close enough to him to know when my children were suffering, and I would know how to help them.

One of my children went through some hard stuff as a teenager. The hardest part was that I did not know how much pain they were in.

By the time I discovered it, they had experienced significant trauma, affecting their mental health. It was heart-wrenching. I had always felt that if you were suffering, all you had to do was be as obedient to God as possible, and things would improve. Somehow, my natural rule-keeping mind had interpreted the gospel I had been taught as transactional. You live a certain way, and you receive specific blessings. I assumed it was as easy as that.

During this same time, our family moved and lost most of the sense of community that I had always found in my religion. I tried to find a new community but felt uncomfortable. I remember consciously thinking, "Well, do I attend church because it is what I believe or because of the friendships there?" I had always thought it was my deep belief system, but when the community was taken away, I realized how much of my attendance had to do with friendships.

I had also always required my children to attend church with me. At one point, I realized the trauma that had caused my struggling child. I saw that there are circumstances when religious practices can be harmful to mental health. That shocked me and seemed contradictory to my transactional gospel belief system. I started to question everything I had previously clung to.

These experiences were a real knock on the head, forcing me to rethink everything I had believed. I stepped back from the religious beliefs that were part of my upbringing and adult life.

I stopped attending church meetings but never stopped praying to the God I had known my entire life. During this time, the most astonishing realization was that I still felt a powerful spiritual connection to God outside my organized religious practices. That was a complete shock to me as I had always thought strict religious rules brought a closeness to God that was impossible otherwise. This realization was liberating. It sent me on a deep soul-searching journey to determine what I believed without anyone telling me what to think. I felt unconstrained to dig deeper into my connections and beliefs than I ever had before.

A quote from M. Scott Peck's book, The Road Less Traveled, comes to mind here:

"To proceed very far through the desert, you must be willing to meet existential suffering and work it through. In order to do this, the attitude toward pain has to change. This happens when we accept that everything that happens to us has been designed for our spiritual growth."

Our hardships can either make us or break us. For some, hardship will be seen as a roadblock, and they will hunker down and stay stagnant. Others will take the hardship and learn what they can to progress. We get to decide our reaction to the hard things that happen to us in life.

During this time of faith growth, I focused more on developing my authentic spirituality than clinging to a religious rulebook. That brought so much liberation for me. I see the many benefits of organized religion, and I wholeheartedly support those who embrace it on their journey. Nevertheless, focusing on my connection to a higher power and a non-judgmental view of different types of spirituality has helped me to feel more at peace. Understanding that your spirituality exists in or outside religion can be liberating and exhilarating and allows you to search deep into your soul to learn to know yourself honestly. My journey continues, and I don't know where it will lead me. But I do know that my current stage allows me to see everyone differently. I realize we are all on our individual journey, and it's not for me to judge another's progress.

One fascinating way to study religion and spirituality is to examine the concept of faith stages. James W. Fowler, an American theologian and professor of theology and human development at Emory University, wrote Stages of Faith: The Psychology of Human Development and the Quest for Meaning. His book describes the faith stages as follows:

Stage 1: Intuitive-Projective Faith – Faith is developed through stories, images, and the influence of others. Fantasy and reality often get mixed together. It involves creating a sense of right and wrong and punishment and reward. This early stage includes magical interpretations of God and the universe.

Stage 2: Mythic-Literal Faith–Faith develops according to the beliefs and stories of one's family and religious group; however, these stories are taken very literally. This stage tends to separate good and evil into rigid categories and see life's tribulations and blessings as a result of choices.

Stage 3: Synthetic-Conventional Faith – One develops an all-encompassing belief system based on their social circles and the ideas their community shares. In this stage, most people's faith and beliefs provide a sense of belonging to a group. The moral structure is based on the expectations of others. One may have difficulty seeing outside the box and realizing they are "inside" a belief system. This stage usually occurs in young adulthood and can carry through into adulthood. Some will stay in this stage for life.

Stage 4: Individuated-Reflective Faith – Authority is relocated to the individual, and people start to see outside the box and realize other boxes exist. While still attuned to other's beliefs and expectations, one can pass the meanings and concepts through an internal filter before accepting them. One begins to demystify previously held stories and symbols to look deeper into logic and explicit meaning. People in other stages may think stage four people have "slipped," but they are actually moving forward.

Stage 5: Conjunctive Faith – It is rare to reach this stage before mid-life. One realizes that truth is more multifaceted and complex and becomes more aware of injustice and division. This results in a desire to broaden spiritual horizons and welcome the truths of different systems, bringing an entirely new dimension to faith. They may return to sacred stories from their past stages but can now see them without being stuck in a theological box.

Stage 6: Universalizing Faith – Very few people are in this phase. It involves a strong sense of universal justice that cuts through national and racial boundaries. It consists in taking action on many new truths learned in stage five and devoting time to suitable causes to improve the world. Fowler mentions Mother Teresa, Martin Luther King, Jr., and Mahatma Gandhi as examples of people in this stage.

Fowler explains how the development of people's spiritual awareness runs parallel to other aspects of human development. Most spiritual growth begins in very immature stages based on basic ideas learned from our parents or society. As we mature, we understand things more logically but view faith as transactional. As we have more spiritual experiences, we may accept our belief system as the only truth. Many people stay in this lower stage forever, operating in an us-versus-them world.

Life hardships challenge some of our thinking in various stages. Through trials, we mature and realize that life is not black and white like some religions preach. Through these challenges, we often feel that the stories we have been telling ourselves no longer make sense.

Deep soul-searching will usually lead us to emerge into Stage 4 faith. We think more critically and rethink some of our former belief systems. Stage 4 can feel disappointing as we question everything we once firmly believed. In his book *Breathing Under Water*, Richard Rohr states, "All mature spirituality, in one sense or another, is about letting go and unlearning."

James Fowler agrees that this "unlearning" is crucial to spiritual growth. It is vital not to stay in Stage 4 forever. It is okay to linger here for a while and take time to analyze values and beliefs. Stage 4 can be a tricky spot and is often referred to as a faith crisis, but it can help us advance to other levels of learning and growth.

One of my favorite concepts in the faith stages journey is to *transcend and include*. As we move through the stages, we can remember everything we learned in the prior phases. As we transcend through the stages, we *should* include the parts that still feel right or resonate as we progress through these further stages. When a person is ready to continue their faith journey after lingering in Stage 4, they should be prepared to include the necessary parts to further their voyage.

Stage 5 faith is eccentric. This stage includes more uncertainty as we realize we do not have all the answers. We often bring many of our previous stages to Stage 5, but we use them differently as we work to find personal answers for our own lives rather than spending time judging what everyone else is doing.

People rarely advance to Stage 6 faith, but we can strive to get there. This type of faith is lived in peace and service to others. People in Stage 6 overwhelmingly accept the divinity of every living thing. They realize that all humans are the same regardless of their belief systems. What a beautiful faith stage to strive for.

This concept of faith stages and spirituality might seem straightforward to some people. However, I am not ashamed to admit that I was in my forties before discovering that religion and spirituality differed. I was stuck in a lower stage of faith and thought of faith as transactional.

Religion and spirituality are separate concepts. One may lead to the other, but they can also stand alone. There is happiness that comes from both. Religion can bring joy from being part of a like-minded tribe that puts its efforts toward helping others. On the other hand, spirituality brings deep inner happiness by focusing on meaning, purpose, and connection.

Research has shown that understanding the differences between religion and spirituality can be healthy. For example, a study published in the *Journal of Health Psychology* found that individuals who identified as "spiritual but not religious" (SBNR) had better mental health outcomes than those who identified as spiritual and religious or as neither spiritual nor religious. The study suggests that SBNR individuals may experience greater well-being because they can explore their spirituality without the constraints of institutionalized religion.[1]

Other research has shown that religion and spirituality can affect health outcomes differently. A study published in the *Journal of Gerontological Social Work* found that spirituality was associated with greater subjective well-being and life satisfaction among older adults. In contrast, religiousness was associated with greater levels of social support and greater involvement in religious activities.[2]

Understanding the difference between religion and spirituality can help promote interfaith dialogue and understanding. A study published in the *Journal of Psychology and Theology* found that individuals with a more nuanced understanding of religion and spirituality were likelier to have positive attitudes toward individuals from different religious backgrounds.[3]

---

1   Kim et al., 2018.

2   Hodge et al., 2003.

3   Wilkinson et al., 2018.

Whether religious or not, take time to find your spirituality, whatever that may be. Find where you feel connections to something greater than you and develop that connection to a deeper level.

What is the essence of your inner self?

Reflect on the core values, beliefs, and principles that define your inner being. Explore how these aspects align with your actions and decisions in daily life. Consider whether there are any inconsistencies and how you can work toward greater alignment.

_____

_____

_____

_____

_____

_____

_____

_____

_____

_____

_____

_____

_____

_____

What role do your relationships play in your spiritual journey?

Reflect on your connections with others and how they impact your spiritual growth. Consider how your interactions and shared experiences contribute to your sense of purpose and fulfillment.

_____

_____

_____

_____

_____

_____

_____

_____

_____

_____

_____

_____

_____

_____

In what ways do you seek transcendent or divine experiences?

Contemplate your pursuit of transcendent or mystical moments in life. Reflect on the practices, rituals, or experiences that allow you to connect with a higher power or deeper spiritual reality. Consider how these moments shape your perspective and provide spiritual insight.

_____

_____

_____

_____

_____

_____

_____

_____

_____

_____

_____

_____

_____

_____

_____

_____

_____

_____

ACTIVITIES FOR WEEK 9:

1. Study the stages of faith by reading *The Stages of Faith* by James W. Fowler or *The Road Less Traveled* by M. Scott Peck.

2. Use meditation to develop your spirituality separate from whatever religion you practice.

Write about your experience doing these activities:

_____

_____

_____

_____

_____

_____

_____

_____

_____

_____

_____

CHAPTER 10:
Find Purpose in Adversity

"Challenge and adversity are meant
to help you know who you are. Storms hit
our weakness but unlock your true strength."
— ROY T. BENNETT, *THE LIGHT IN THE HEART*

As a teenager, my family moved two thousand miles from the only community I had ever known to a place I knew nothing about. I was thirteen, and my dad had an opportunity to attend school on the other side of the country. I had spent my entire life in the same place where I felt safe.

Thirteen is not the most secure age, and leaving my home to enter a new school and meet new friends took much work. Everyone around me seemed so confident, and I felt like an oddball. I was from a white, Christian, homogenous town and moved to a diverse city with new experiences, slang, clothing, and cultures. I was a fish out of water, and it took me months to acclimate. I was a quiet, insecure, narrow-minded, and inexperienced girl from a state most of my new peers had never heard of. I had to learn to be brave and reach out to people whom I wanted to get to know better.

At first, I waited for others to reach out to me, but I soon realized I had to be the one to reach out. I had to learn to be friendly and take the risk of talking to people to try to make friends. I had never experienced that before, and it was tough. I eventually found friendships through school and church and learned to appreciate and embrace people different from me. I learned so much about myself and others through that time. I gained confidence, and I learned empathy for those who may be outsiders. When our time there was over, and we moved back home to our original community, that was no picnic either. I was sad to leave my newfound friendships but excited to see my friends at home. When I arrived, I found they had moved on without me a bit, and I once again found myself trying to fit in.

Skip forward to a young married person hoping for my own family. My husband and I married young and waited six years before we felt ready for children. By then, we were ready and excited about that new adventure. When I finally became pregnant, we were so excited that we told everyone. At eleven weeks (about two and a half months), I started bleeding, and within a week, I had miscarried.

It was one of the most painful experiences in my life. The experience alone was emotional and heartbreaking. However, I constantly had to explain what had happened because we had told so many people. I wanted to hide in my house and not go anywhere. I was so confused about why it happened and extremely sad. We tried again as soon as we could, and again I miscarried. Miscarriage is always heartbreaking, but because we had no children, it also brought the worry of being unable to carry to full-term.

The third pregnancy was stressful. We waited until I was almost five months before we told anyone out of fear of it happening again. However, I carried that beautiful baby girl to full term. She was healthy and brought us more joy than we ever imagined.

After that, we experienced another miscarriage, infertility requiring surgery, and a high-risk twin pregnancy ending with five weeks of bed rest and an early but safe delivery.

From there, I had an unexpected pregnancy that ended in miscarriage.

After that, a high-risk pregnancy with six weeks of bed rest before delivering six weeks early.

Our childbearing years were one long roller coaster ride that ended with four healthy, happy, unique humans in our family. Through all those experiences, I learned that I could do hard things, that I do not always have control over what happens, and that the best blessings sometimes come with the most challenging life experiences.

On top of these challenges, I have faced the heartache of raising teenagers, the confusion of faith transitions, the sorrow of my mother's passing, the despair of watching a sister struggle with addiction, and the helplessness of supporting my husband as he navigates the emotional toll of complicated family relationships. Let's face it, trials suck. However, they also bring more growth and freedom to your life if you embrace the lessons and lean on those you love for support. You will learn more about yourself and your strength, relationships, and other people and more about life and wisdom than you have ever wanted to learn. Furthermore, if you understand these things, you will look back with gratitude because you will know that it made you stronger.

As a child, I had so many fears. I worried to no end about the "what-ifs" of life. However, the more trials I experienced and the more I survived, the less I feared. I realized that I was stronger than I gave myself credit for and that I had a tribe and a support system who would help me. It also made me want to be that tribe and support system for others. I went from being fearful of life to embracing all the messiness of it, knowing that strength comes not from being comfortable but from leaning into the uncomfortable and looking for the lessons to be learned rather than the experiences to be feared.

The notion that hardships in life contribute to personal growth and resilience is a well-established concept in psychology and human development. A study conducted by Tedeschi and Calhoun in 2004, titled "Posttraumatic Growth: Conceptual Foundations and Empirical Evidence," explores how individuals can experience positive psychological changes after enduring traumatic events. The research suggests that facing and overcoming adversity can increase psychological strength, greater appreciation for life, and a more profound sense of meaning.

Another relevant article by Masten emphasizes the resilience of individuals in the face of adversity.[1] Masten's work highlights how adversity can prompt individuals to develop coping mechanisms, adaptability, and problem-solving skills, ultimately making them more resilient.

This research supports that life's hardships can equip us to endure future situations with more wisdom, grace, humility, and strength. They emphasize the potential for personal growth and positive psychological changes often resulting from facing and overcoming adversity.

Hardships come in all shapes and sizes. Trials bring growth. We cannot compare the trials that we experience to the trials of others. We are unique and will experience and react to things in diverse ways.

---

1   "Ordinary Magic: Resilience Processes in Development," 2001.

What lessons can you learn from your challenges?

Reflect on your specific challenges and identify valuable lessons or insights from them. Consider how these lessons can contribute to your personal growth and resilience.

_____

_____

_____

_____

_____

_____

_____

What are your sources of support?

Consider the people, resources, or support networks available during your challenges. Reflect on how you can lean on these sources of support to help you navigate and cope with your trials.

_____

_____

_____

_____

_____

_____

_____

_____

How can you reframe your perspective?

Consider whether there are alternative ways to view your situation. Explore how changing your perspective or mindset about your challenges can empower you to find strength and adapt more effectively.

_____

_____

_____

_____

_____

_____

_____

_____

_____

_____

_____

_____

_____

_____

_____

_____

ACTIVITIES FOR WEEK 10:

1. Engage in mindfulness meditation practices. This activity involves paying focused, non-judgmental attention to the present moment. Regular mindfulness meditation can enhance emotional regulation, reduce stress, and increase your ability to bounce back from challenges.

2. Start or continue a journal to express thoughts and emotions. This can be a powerful tool for building resilience. Writing down your experiences, feelings, and thoughts allows for self-reflection and can help you gain clarity and perspective on challenging situations. It can also track personal growth over time.

3. Identify your support group. Choose those who have a positive outlook on life and who love you for who you are. Sharing your challenges and seeking emotional support with the right people can help alleviate stress and provide a sense of belonging.

Write about your experience doing these activities:

_____

_____

_____

_____

CHAPTER 11:
Look for Opportunities to Grow

"It is only possible to live happily ever after on a daily basis."
— MARGARET BONANNO

Maintaining a positive outlook and actively seeking the good in our daily experiences can significantly enhance our inner peace and happiness.

Once at work, I was overlooked for a big promotion. It was a new position created with many of my job duties. Because the job description included many things I had been doing for years, I assumed it was a promotion I would quickly get. When the company selected someone else, it was a shock and, frankly, hurtful. I spent much time questioning my value to the company and whether I should stay. I eventually decided to stay. I did vast amounts of self-reflection during that time. I realized I had to focus on what I could control: how well I did my job and how I treated others. So, I started working even harder with the parts of my job that were left, and I found joy. It probably took me longer than I want to admit getting over it, but when I did, I realized I was left with the parts of my job that I enjoyed. I also learned more about myself, my priorities, and my work relationships through this experience.

I have had many heart-aching, confusing experiences. I am not always great at finding perspective, but I usually get there at some point. I have learned that leaning into uncomfortable situations and painful experiences is essential.

Lean in and allow yourself to feel all of the emotions. Take time to mourn, be sad, or feel anger. Those are normal human responses. Admit that you feel them, ponder why, and share your feelings with those you trust. Just do not linger too long on those unpleasant emotions. The lessons and enlightenment start to come when you move into seeking a broader perspective and understanding. Sometimes, this can feel like a roller coaster ride as you go from adverse emotions to perspective and back to feeling unhappiness again. Do not worry. It is all part of the healing process.

I am at a point in my life where I am trying to lean into the uncomfortable to find growth. Cold plunges are a trend right now. Scientific research has shown that submerging yourself in a pool of cold water (below sixty degrees Fahrenheit) for at least three minutes can improve your mental health, energize you, and improve your metabolism, among other benefits. I have always had an aversion to cold water. I will only get in a swimming pool if it is sunny and over eighty degrees. I attempted a cold plunge because I have been trying to embrace the uncomfortable.

It was *so cold*. However, I could withstand it and found that while it was unpleasant, it was doable. Research also shows that turning your shower water on cold for the last thirty seconds of your shower will provide the same benefits. I *never* thought I would be able to do that. I *hate* cold water. However, I did it, and it was uncomfortable. I was doing it to prove I could embrace the uncomfortable more than for the health benefits. That is a frivolous example, but things that make you stretch or move out of your comfort zone can open your mind and bring growth. Find your version of a cold plunge that makes you step out of your comfort zone.

I am naturally quite introverted and have a work-first, play-later personality. Sometimes, I have something to accomplish in my job, and someone will want to come to my office for a chat. I must remind myself to stop, breathe, and listen to learn more about the person and their situation. It does not come naturally to me. I enjoy work friendships and getting to know others, but my internal drive to be productive haunts me. However, when I take the time to chat with others, I enjoy my job more and learn to appreciate the people around me. Stepping out of my comfort zone brings growth and happiness.

If you are intentional about it, you will find life lessons and growth in your daily experiences. Be curious about the world, seek to understand others, and be kind. These three things done daily can significantly improve your happiness and inner peace.

Numerous studies have shown that a positive outlook on life contributes to greater emotional well-being.

For instance, in their research, Lyubomirsky, King, and Diener (2005) found that individuals who habitually engage in positive thinking and gratitude exercises tend to report higher life satisfaction and happiness levels. This indicates that consciously focusing on the positive aspects of life can directly impact your overall well-being.

Scholarly research in positive psychology supports the notion that maintaining a positive outlook and actively seeking the good in daily experiences can improve inner peace and happiness. These practices enhance emotional well-being and offer practical strategies for individuals to nurture a more positive and fulfilling life.

I remind myself often that happiness is a choice. I also know that happiness is different for everyone. You, my friend, are the only one who can determine where your happiness lies. This book is meant to be a journey to lead you to those conclusions. Seek happiness and peace as you go about your daily life.

Happiness comes from our reactions to our daily experiences. You can choose to see the blessings and the lessons or the challenges and the failures. It is up to you. Perspective is the most essential part of inner peace.

What small moments in your daily life bring you joy?
Reflect on the simple, everyday occurrences that make you smile or feel content. It could be savoring a cup of coffee in the morning, a friendly greeting from a colleague, or a beautiful sunset.

_____

_____

_____

_____

_____

_____

_____

_____

_____

_____

_____

_____

_____

Are there any habits or routines that detract from your daily happiness?

Take a close look at your daily routines and behaviors. Are there any habits that consistently bring negativity or stress? Identifying them is the first step toward making positive changes.

_____

_____

_____

_____

_____

_____

_____

_____

_____

_____

_____

_____

_____

_____

_____

_____

_____

_____

ACTIVITIES FOR WEEK 11:

1. Keep a daily journal where you reflect on your experiences, emotions, and thoughts. Writing down your daily interactions and challenges can provide valuable insights over time. It allows you to identify recurring patterns, areas of personal growth, and opportunities for improvement.

2. Actively seek feedback from trusted friends, colleagues, or mentors. Constructive feedback can help you gain different perspectives on your actions and behaviors. It provides self-improvement and growth opportunities by addressing blind spots or areas where you may not be fully aware of your impact on others.

3. Lean into something uncomfortable this week. It may be turning your shower on cold for thirty seconds or conversing with someone different. Nevertheless, whatever it is, it should make you squirm a bit.

Write about your experience doing these activities:

_____

_____

_____

_____

CHAPTER 12:
Reflect on Your Progress

"Without reflection, we go blindly on our way, creating more unintended consequences and failing to achieve anything useful."
— **MARGARET J. WHEATLEY**

This book provides a journey of self-reflection through accepting yourself, connecting with others, and embracing the unknown to help you find more happiness and inner peace. Whether you skimmed it or read it slowly and reflectively, I hope you found some tools to help you work toward a fulfilled life.

As I have mentioned many times throughout the book, it has been a lifelong quest of mine to master each of these tools. I have yet to reach that point. I am a work in progress, but growth does come when I repeatedly focus on them. I am constantly working toward accepting myself and living my truth. I still struggle to connect with others sometimes, but I keep trying. I am growing and learning by working to embrace the unknown every day. I tell you this in hopes that you will remember that the principles in this book are part of a lifelong journey. You most likely will only be able to do some of these things after some time. The goal is to continually focus on these principles, forgive yourself when you mess up, and keep working.

Self-reflection is an invaluable tool on the path to personal progress and growth. Taking the time to introspect and assess your experiences, thoughts, and actions allows you to gain deeper insights into yourself and your life. It serves as a compass, guiding you better to understand your goals, values, and aspirations. Through self-reflection, you can identify areas where improvement is needed, recognize patterns of behavior that may be hindering your progress, and celebrate your successes, no matter how small. It is a process that fosters self-awareness and self-empowerment, enabling you to make informed choices, set meaningful goals, and ultimately become the architect of your personal development journey. In a world filled with constant distractions and external influences, the ability to pause, reflect, and chart our course is a crucial skill that empowers us to lead more intentional and fulfilling lives.

I have learned to find happiness and inner peace through practicing these principles and self-reflecting. I am constantly working on this and have never mastered the concepts. However, I am different today than when I began my journey for happiness. I can forgive myself and love myself through my many imperfections. I am constantly curious rather than judgmental. Because I aim to be non-judgmental, I can connect with others on a deeper level, especially those whose ideas differ from mine. Having people in my life who are different from me has helped me to more fully embrace the unknown and lean into and be curious about things that feel uncomfortable to me. This all started as a quest for happiness, and in turn, I have found so much growth.

You can research each one of the subjects discussed in this book on your own. Google Scholar will provide hundreds of scholarly articles. You can listen to the stories of others and consider your own stories. You can reflect on the many lessons and do the work to learn the necessary skills. Furthermore, now that you have started that journey, keep it up. Every. Single. Day

SELF-REFLECTION QUESTIONS:

Part 1: Accept Yourself

How have you applied the concept of authenticity in your life, and what impact has it had on your relationships and overall well-being?

_____

_____

_____

_____

_____

_____

_____

_____

_____

_____

_____

_____

_____

_____

_____

_____

What values and principles have you identified as your core character traits, and how can you continue aligning your actions with these principles daily?

_____

_____

_____

_____

_____

_____

_____

How have you embraced your imperfections as part of your unique journey toward happiness and personal growth, and how can you cultivate self-compassion?

_____

_____

_____

_____

_____

_____

_____

_____

What aspects of your life have you approached with curiosity and a growth mindset, and how have these inquiries led to personal development and happiness?

_____

_____

_____

_____

_____

_____

_____

Part 2: Connect with Others

Reflect on the importance of friendships in your life. How have you strengthened or built new friendships, and how can you nurture these connections?

_____

_____

_____

_____

_____

_____

_____

How have you improved your ability to communicate your needs and establish healthy boundaries? What steps can you take to maintain and further develop these skills?

_____

_____

_____

_____

_____

_____

Reflect on a recent situation where you were tempted to participate in gossip. What alternative actions or responses could you have taken to promote a more positive and constructive conversation?

_____

_____

_____

_____

_____

_____

_____

Share instances when seeking out diverse perspectives enriched your understanding and decision-making. How can you incorporate this practice more consistently?

_____

_____

_____

_____

_____

_____

_____

Part 3: Embrace the Unknown

What aspects of inner spirituality have resonated with you, and how have they contributed to your inner peace and happiness? How can you continue to cultivate this aspect of your life?

_____

_____

_____

_____

_____

_____

_____

_____

Describe how you have integrated the idea of finding growth opportunities in everyday experiences. What strategies can you employ to continue this practice?

_____

_____

_____

_____

_____

_____

_____

_____

_____

_____

_____

_____

_____

_____

_____

_____

_____

Conclusion

Based on what you have learned in this book, what specific actions or changes would you like to implement to foster ongoing happiness and growth?

_____

_____

_____

_____

_____

_____

_____

_____

_____

_____

_____

_____

_____

_____

_____

_____

References

Chapter 1:

Chopra, Deepak MD, and Sarah Platt-Finger (2023). *Living in the Light*. Harmony Books, 2021. 51.

Sheldon, K. M., Ryan, R. M., & Reis, H. T. (1996). "What makes for a good day? Competence and autonomy in the day and the person." *Personality and Social Psychology Bulletin*, 22(12), 1270-1279.

Wood, A. M., Linley, P. A., Maltby, J., Kashdan, T. B., & Hurling, R. (2011). "Using personal and psychological strengths leads to increases in well-being over time: A longitudinal study and the development of the strengths use questionnaire." *Personality and Individual Differences*, 50(1), 15-19.

Chapter 2:

Fiske, Susan T. "Stereotype content: Warmth and competence endure." *Journal of Social Issues*, vol. 63, no. 4, 2017, 878-899. https://journals.sagepub.com/doi/full/10.1177/0963721417738825.

The Decision Lab: https://thedecisionlab.com/reference-guide/psychology/stereotypes

Chapter 3:

Kashdan, T. B., & Rottenberg, J. (2010). "Psychological flexibility as a fundamental aspect of health." *Clinical Psychology Review*, 30(7), 865-878.

Neff, K. D., & Beretvas, S. N. (2013). "The role of self-compassion in romantic relationships." *Self and Identity*, 12(1), 78-98.

Chapter 5:
Demir, M., Ozdemir, M., Weitekamp, L. A., & Boysan, M. (2011). "I am so happy because today I found my friend: Friendship and personality as predictors of happiness." *Journal of Happiness Studies*, 12(2), 289-302.

Gable, S. L., Reis, H. T., Impett, E. A., & Asher, E. R. (2004). "What do you do when things go right? The intrapersonal and interpersonal benefits of sharing positive events." *Journal of Personality and Social Psychology*, 87(2), 228-245.

Kawachi, I., & Berkman, L. F. (2001). "Social ties and mental health." *Journal of Urban Health*, 78(3), 458-467.

Chapter 6:
Michie, S., Abraham, C., Whittington, C., McAteer, J., & Gupta, S. (2011). "Effective techniques in healthy eating and physical activity interventions: A meta-regression." *Health Psychology*, 30(4), 520–529.

Rotter, J. B. (1966). "Generalized expectancies for internal versus external control of reinforcement." *Psychological Monographs: General and Applied*, 80(1), 1-28.

Chapter 7:
Seligman, M. "Positive psychology: A field in its infancy." *American Psychologist*, Vol. 55, No. 1, 2000, 5-14.

Sonja Lyubomirsky, King, L., & Diener, E. "The benefits of frequent positive affect: Does happiness lead to success?" *Psychological Bulletin*, Vol. 131, No. 6, 2005, 803-855.

Fredrickson, B. F. "The broaden-and-build theory of positive emotions." *Philosophical Transactions of the Royal Society B: Biological Sciences*, Vol. 359, No. 1449, 2004, 1367-1378.

Chapter 8:

Levine, J. M., & Moreland, R. L. (1994). "Group socialization: Theory and research." In M. A. Hogg & D. J. Terry (Eds.), *Social identity processes in organizational contexts*. Sage Publications. 143-170.

Malka, A., Lelkes, Y., Srivastava, S. B., & Cohen, A. B. (2010). The association of religiosity and political conservatism: The role of political engagement. *Political Psychology*, 31(5), 727-754.

Richard, O. C., Murthi, B. P. S., & Ismail, K. M. (2007). "The impact of racial and gender diversity in management on financial performance: A generalization." *Journal of Business Research*, 60(3), 273-281.

Page, S. E. (2007). "The difference: How the power of diversity creates better groups, firms, schools, and societies." Princeton University Press.

Oviedo-Trespalacios, O., Haque, M. M., & King, M. (2019). "Diversity and inclusion for innovation: A critical review and future research agenda." SAGE Open, 9(2), 2158244019845520.

Chapter 9:

Fowler, J. W. *Stages of Faith: The Psychology of Human Development and the Quest for Meaning*. HarperCollins, 1981.

Hodge, D. R., Horvath, V. E., & Kim, S. Y. (2003). "Religion and spirituality: Linkages to physical health." *Journal of Gerontological Social Work*, 39(3-4), 19-35.

Kim, J. H., Lee, J. E., & Sung, K. (2018). "Spiritual and religious self-identification and mental health outcomes in Korea: A nation-wide cross-sectional study." *Journal of Health Psychology*, 23(7), 909-919.

Peck, M. Scott MD. *The Road Less Traveled*. Simon & Schuster, 1978.

Wilkinson, M., Roebuck, A., & Thomas, G. (2018). "Religion, spirituality, and interfaith dialogue: The significance of developing a nuanced understanding." *Journal of Psychology and Theology*, 46(4), 257-268.

Chapter 10:

Matsen, A. S. (2001). "Ordinary magic: Resilience processes in development. American Psychologist, 56(3), 227-238. doi:10.1037//0003-066x.56.3.227.

Tedeschi, R. G., & Calhoun, L. G. (2004). "Posttraumatic growth: Conceptual foundations and empirical evidence." Psychological Inquiry, 15(1), 1-18. Taylor & Francis, Ltd.

Chapter 11:

Lyubomirsky, S., & King, L. (2005). "The benefits of frequent positive affect: Does happiness lead to success?" Psychological Bulletin, American Psychological Association, 131(6), 803-855.

About the Author

Alison has a passion for education and personal development. A life-long educator, she has taught adults and children and is currently working in higher education in Utah. With a love for writing, reading, and spending time with her family, Alison finds joy exploring themes of happiness, inner peace, and perspective. Her interest in psychology fuels her desire to understand human behavior and interactions. Alison's work is driven by a deep-seated desire to empower others to welcome joy into their lives.